W0232941

365 DAYS OF
self-care

DAILY GUIDANCE FOR
GREATER WELL-BEING

Chris Spriggs

365 DAYS OF SELF-CARE

An Hachette UK Company
www.hachette.co.uk

Vie Books, an imprint of Summersdale Publishers
Part of Octopus Publishing Group Limited
Carmelite House
50 Victoria Embankment
LONDON
EC4Y 0DZ
UK

www.summersdale.com

The authorized representative in the EEA is Hachette Ireland, 8 Castlecourt Centre, Dublin 15, D15 XTP3, Ireland (email: info@hbgi.ie)

Printed and bound in China

ISBN: 978-1-83799-705-3
eISBN: 978-1-83799-706-0

This FSC® label means that materials and other controlled sources used for the product have been responsibly sourced

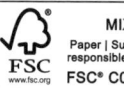

MIX
Paper | Supporting responsible forestry
FSC® C016973

Substantial discounts on bulk quantities of Summersdale books are available to corporations, professional associations and other organizations. For details contact general enquiries: telephone: +44 (0) 1243 771107 or email: enquiries@summersdale.com

Disclaimer
Neither the author nor the publisher can be held responsible for any injury, loss or claim – be it health, financial or otherwise – arising out of the use, or misuse, of the suggestions made herein. This book is not intended as a substitute for the medical advice of a doctor or physician. If you are experiencing problems with your physical or mental health, it is always best to follow the advice of a medical professional.

To ....

From ....

introduction

Welcome to this book of uplifting, daily self-care tips. Maybe self-care sounds selfish, expensive and time-consuming, but self-care is 1 per cent luxury and 99 per cent necessity. Investing even a little time in self-care can boost your mood, reduce stress and improve your sleep and health. Self-care means nurturing an attitude of kindness towards yourself. This loving attitude is expressed through small, regular acts that take care of your well-being.

Modern life includes many distractions, expectations and pressures, so it becomes easy to forget that you are worthy of care, just as you are. *365 Days of Self-Care* is practical, relational and spiritual. Through short daily entries (think of

them as friendly nudges) you will discover things you can do, and not do, to support your self-caring capacity. Some tips are intended to immediately benefit your sleep, nutritional choices, money, movement and relationships. There are also inspirational quotes to reset your perspective that may open up new ways of being "you" in the world.

The intention of this book is to weave self-care into everyday life. Go with whatever serves you, leave aside what doesn't. As you care for yourself and grow in self-love and acceptance, so this capacity radiates out to others, near and far. Ultimately, this book is an invitation to experience being a precious expression of life itself, fully worthy of care.

january

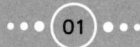

Notice the gift of being alive right now, even as you read these words. Feel the air in your nostrils as you breathe in. Notice the gentle sound as you breathe out. This is a brand new day. You are here!

Today, go for a walk (or bicycle ride) to somewhere you can enjoy a quiet view, perhaps to look across a field, down from a hilltop or along a river. Being in open natural space provides a larger visual perspective, which is relaxing for your eyes and grounds your body in the present moment.

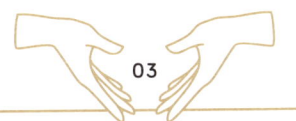

03

Success is liking yourself, liking what you do, and liking how you do it.

MAYA ANGELOU

•••(04)•••

Rather than rushing at the start of the day, when you wake notice your breathing and the weight of the duvet on your body. Notice where your body feels coolest and where it feels warmest. Listen to the sounds around you. This tunes you into your body from the outset rather than letting anxious thoughts rush in and take charge.

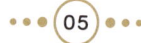

Make your home a place that shows you matter! What clutter needs to be cleared out? Do this today. What items bring you comfort? Whether it is beautiful plants, cherished photographs, inspiring art or soft cushions, have them at hand or easy to see.

Today, don't try to make every moment count; this is far too much pressure for anyone. Easing back occasionally isn't laziness – it's a way of pacing yourself in a frenetic world. Read, watch or listen to something that restores you or puts a smile on your face. Enjoy yourself.

••• 07 •••

Ask your friends what they think you already do well in terms of self-care. Be open to being surprised with a fresh challenge from people you trust.

Do some basic exercises to invigorate your body and mind. Press-ups will strengthen your arms, shoulders and core. Squeezing your glutes (bottom muscles) as you do it will add another layer. You don't need fancy equipment for this. Begin with doing five or ten, keeping it within a comfortable range before adding more. Little and often is the best approach.

Exercise activates a symphony of brain chemicals, including dopamine, throughout the whole body, creating the feeling of motivation. Why not do ten star jumps or a minute of invisible skipping (skipping without a rope!) just to wake up your body? Or just move your body in whatever way it chooses – it knows what it likes!

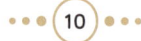

Smell is a powerful way of evoking positive memories. Introduce a pleasing scent with joyful associations into your home, or consider something you can take with you on the go; this might be a scented candle, a spice, a plant or a certain food.

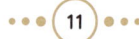

Have an alcohol-free week. An occasional drink with an evening meal or with friends might feel relaxing, but alcohol is a depressant that prevents the body from absorbing the amino acid tryptophan, which has a vital role in regulating mood. Having a break from alcohol may improve your sleep and hydration.

The only journey is the one within.

RAINER MARIA RILKE

How are you feeling right now? You don't need to judge yourself, whether your mood is pleasant or low; just notice how you are. Can you describe the feeling in one or two words? This practice develops your ability to slow down and notice emotions, strengthening your capacity to self-regulate and feel more in tune with yourself. By doing this, you are less likely to get caught up in other people's dramas.

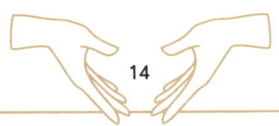

Love yourself first, and everything else falls in line. You really have to love yourself to get anything done in this world.

LUCILLE BALL

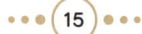

Enjoying time outside without striving to get somewhere can be good for your physical and mental well-being. Being outdoors helps regulate your sleep-wake cycle, which reduces feelings of exhaustion. Exposure to daylight also gives you vitamin D, activating the brain chemical serotonin, which promotes positive moods. A vitamin D supplement is an additional option.

A healthy self-care routine doesn't have to include elaborate or expensive activities (although it can if you choose). Simple, daily practices often make more of a difference than "one big thing", for example, including foods in your breakfast that support good gut health, such as yogurt, oats or avocado.

Play a piece of music that brings back happy memories for you. Music is a wonderful way of elevating energy. If you want to, why not dance or sing along? Doing this releases chemicals in the body that boost mood and motivation, helping you to shake off tension.

Try this experiment: for a week, jot down at least one positive from your day, every day, and write down why this thing is positive for you. Harvesting the good moments present in your life by writing them down will influence your perception of the world and help you tap into your resilience.

**Just for today, allow yourself
to embrace all that you are
every moment. Know that
you are a vessel of light.**

IYANLA VANZANT

If you feel upset or troubled today, rather
than squash the feeling or deny it, bring some
tenderness towards your experience, just like a
caring parent does with a child. Place your hand
over your heart (or wherever you feel the emotion
in your body) and speak a soothing sentence, for
example, "It's okay, I'm here."

Don't leave good times from the past behind. Find a photograph from a while ago that makes you smile or laugh. Have this image as a screensaver, even just for a day. Connect today with that joyful moment back then.

Smile at a stranger. Whether you are walking down the road, in a shop or on public transport, if it seems appropriate, show someone a happy face. Smiling is contagious and has a positive effect on your own and others' well-being.

Brightening your home or workplace with fresh flowers or attractive plants can lift your mood. Make your flowers last longer by putting a tablespoon of sugar in the water and recutting the stems every two days.

Catch yourself when you are getting worked up. Maybe your mind is going over a situation, or you are feeling frustrated at something beyond your control. Remind yourself that it's time to let it go. A solution is more likely to occur when you are able to think and communicate clearly than when you are in an agitated state of mind.

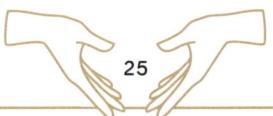

25

Change your thoughts and you change your world.

NORMAN VINCENT PEALE

Managing your money is an important self-care habit because it can help ensure you have some choice about how you use your resources. If you have worries about money, speak to someone you trust, and research what help is available local to where you are.

Mindfulness is an important aspect of self-care. It teaches that when you accept the present moment as it is, including anything that is uncomfortable or difficult, you suffer less. It invites you to stop trying to control everything and focus on the here and now, which is less mentally exhausting.

••• (28) •••

Because of your smile, you make life more beautiful.

THÍCH NHẤT HẠNH

••• (29) •••

Look in the mirror and smile at what you see, then exaggerate your smile. Turn the volume on your smile right up to the maximum. Stretching your facial muscles in this way releases tension, and it is a good way to remember that you are a beautiful person too!

Notice your posture today. How do you typically sit, stand or walk? Do you slouch as if carrying the weight of the world on your shoulders? Does your body become knotted up? Right now, notice how you are sitting or standing. Improve your posture by lifting your chin and nudging your shoulders back.

Self-care is an integral way of life in countries where people report feeling the happiest. The Danish concept *hygge* (see also p.22) is about creating atmospheres and experiences that nourish you rather than focusing on material things. Look around your room. What might energize the atmosphere where you are?

february

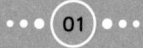

Restore a helpful routine that has been forgotten. Is there something you do that anchors you in feeling safe and connected to the world? It could be something as simple as opening the curtains in the morning and greeting the day. Positive routines can reduce the feeling of being overwhelmed by providing comfort, familiarity and structure.

Use your senses to ground you. Notice three things you can see, three things you can hear and three things you can touch or hold. Tuning into your senses activates the parasympathetic nervous system, strengthening your capacity to self-regulate and reducing anxiety and stress.

Notice textures you enjoy — perhaps fabrics, cushions or objects that are pleasant to hold or be next to. Keep one of these close to you today. Experiencing physical comfort in this way enables the relentless cycle of thinking to settle, leading to a clearer mind.

As you complete a task today — whether it's washing dishes, folding clothes or emptying the bin — don't rush through it. Instead, notice how these ordinary activities are an expression of care. You are inseparable from your environment. As you care for it, so you are caring for yourself.

Learning about a different way of seeing the world that you didn't grow up with can stimulate your curiosity and give you an appreciation of your own and others' perspectives. Find out about a faith, philosophy or concept that is unfamiliar, for example, the Danish concept of *hygge* (meaning "comfort, cosiness and conviviality") or the Chinese philosophy of *Yang Sheng* (which means "to nourish life").

Have a screen-free evening. What would you prefer to do instead? Listen to music, play chess, have a relaxing bath? The screens will be right where you left them afterwards. Giving your body a break from constant stimuli can help you feel more rested.

Those in a hurry do not arrive.

ZEN PROVERB

Bring a new plant into your home. Whether you prefer attractive flowers or a plant with stylish leaves, add life to a corner of your home or a window sill. House plants usually only require a little bit of care now and then yet brighten up a room every day.

What did you enjoy doing as a child that you could revisit: writing stories, foraging, climbing, designing or building things? Be open to these again. Fun is a fabulous expression of self-care, opening up positive new ways of being you in the world.

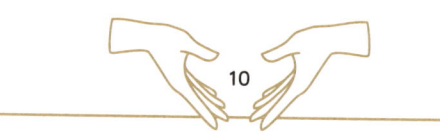

Your self-worth is determined by you. You don't have to depend on someone telling you who you are.

BEYONCÉ

Mental health is a key part of self-care. It is natural for the mind to tighten up around a disappointment or regret and become occupied by negative feelings. But this pulls you out of the real world. Bring awareness to your breathing, body sensations and external sounds. Expanding the space around your thoughts in this way makes problems easier to process and, in time, will make it easier for you to know how to respond.

Exercise is vital for good self-care, mental health and sleep. Aim for at least 30 minutes of exercise you enjoy, three times a week (depending on your health and mobility). Whenever possible, exercise earlier in the day to minimize interference with sleep patterns.

Go for a walk and listen to a podcast as you go. Choose a podcast that matches the length of time you would like to walk, be it 20 minutes or an hour. Perhaps you fancy a comedy, something historical or maybe current affairs. Taking your mind and body for a walk will help your physical and mental health.

Enjoy your own body and notice what is pleasurable for you – you don't need anyone else's permission. Showing appropriate affection with others releases the hormone oxytocin, creating feelings of care, nurture and connection. Hugs, holding hands or a back rub are great ways of showing affection.

Synchronicity is when meaningful coincidences seem to occur in your life without an obvious explanation or just by chance. Pay attention today to the way in which life might be guiding you about a positive direction you need to go in. This might be repeatedly hearing a word or song you were already thinking about, or someone who was on your mind getting in touch with you.

Repairing relationships is an important self-care skill because sometimes relationships rupture through misunderstanding or tiredness. Knowing how to repair them builds your confidence and reduces distress. If your relationship is a healthy one, saying, "I'm sorry *that*..." is more effective than "I'm sorry *if*..."

Life is always changing but you have more resilience than you think. Remember a time when you faced a challenge and overcame it successfully? What did you do? Who did you talk to? How did it feel to take action? Self-care means staying in contact with your own capability.

Today, treat yourself and do something indulgent just for you. This doesn't have to mean spending money – you might like to go for a leisurely walk, research something that fascinates you or watch a film series you can lose yourself in.

Do you have a habit that you know isn't helping you? This isn't about a guilt trip but caring about yourself enough to be honest and aware. Maybe today it is enough just to notice this tendency and be curious about it.

Consider what you're striving for, and what is so important about the goal. Are you just chasing something because everyone else seems to be? You may find that stepping back allows more clarity and insight, enabling you to hone your focus.

"Count your blessings" is an old saying. Go ahead, say them out loud. Include the easy-to-miss things, such as having fresh water from a tap, warmth in your home, people who care about you. Discover how many blessings are already present in your life.

How can you care for yourself if you are always in a rush? Walk somewhere at half your normal pace. Start with walking down the stairs at half-speed. Stretch it to a ten-minute slow walk outdoors sometime. Notice if you feel resistance, an impulse to hurry up. Self-care requires some slowing down, so you can be aware, appreciate the present and connect meaningfully with others.

Do you give yourself permission to occasionally have a good cry? Crying releases toxins and lowers stress hormones and so is actually a helpful self-care practice. Studies suggest that the purpose of crying is to restore your connection with others through mirror neurons in the brain, and it supports the brain's capacity to think clearly.

If you feel you need a positivity boost, try this "mental looking" exercise:

- Look back at how far you have come.

- Look out for who can help you.

- Look around for inspiration and ideas.

- Look within at your own strengths, credibility and experience.

- Now look ahead and consider your next step.

Experiment with eating new fruits or vegetables to nourish yourself. Personal tastes will vary, but beans, seeds, nuts and leafy greens all provide magnesium, which is good for bone and heart health and for regulating your blood pressure.

Try a journal exercise today, for example, who do you admire and why? It might include people you know personally, work colleagues or well-known characters. People who inspire you can bring out your best qualities.

Treat yourself to a manicure or pedicure. A gentle hand or foot rub can be a relaxing treat, and it is a good way of stimulating blood flow in your body, which promotes healing and reduces stress.

If there is a physical ailment that has been bothering you, choose to be brave and arrange to see your local doctor. It is easy to put things off and make excuses, but if something can be done to reduce your discomfort or anxiety, now is the time. Take some positive action towards wellness today.

Remember to stay hydrated, even in colder months. Drinking a sufficient amount of water, around six to eight small glasses a day, enables your body to recover from colds and coughs more quickly. Every cell, tissue and organ in your body depends upon water to function properly, so give them the best chance to work efficiently for you.

march

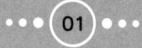

Listen to the birds. Can you detect different types of birdsong? Which sounds are closest, and which are further away? Listening to birds is a way to interrupt your own thoughts with a pleasurable distraction, since their sound is external, unpredictable and often melodic and interesting to listen to.

Spring will be on its way shortly! What could you clean in preparation? Whether it's banging dust from your doormats against a wall, vacuuming the interior of your vehicle or washing flowerpots in the garden, great satisfaction can be gained from revitalizing your environment after winter.

Give different aspects of your well-being a score from 0–10, where 0 is "terrible" and 10 is "great". There is no right or wrong score – low numbers are allowed. Use the number scale to score your sleep, hydration levels, exercise and diet. Whatever score you give, consider how you might improve it by one or two points today.

Take comfort in the words of your favourite authors. Whether it is poetry, literature, philosophy or sci-fi novels, let yourself be inspired by others' imagination. Is there a particular poem or story you have enjoyed over the years that you can recall? Reconnect with it. Memorize a quote that resonates with you.

Self-care means being aware of what you need and having ways to meet that need. Self-care is relevant to everyone. Be a self-care advocate today by talking about it with others, offering suggestions and inviting ideas from others.

Choose positivity today. Obsessing about problems becomes draining – instead, ask yourself what is *not* the problem? For example, what is going well for you and why? What is no longer a worry? Stay with these things and feel the truth of them.

Wash your bed linen and, when you get into bed, take a moment to enjoy the fresh smell of clean sheets. Savour the moment. Not only can this be comforting for your senses but it also helps you to appreciate a household task well done.

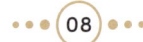

Self-care isn't just a list of pampering actions; it's a way of relating to yourself with gentleness, kindness and respect. What advice would you give to a close friend? Would you tell them to stop caring for themselves so much? Self-care means being a best friend to yourself today.

Every minute life begins all over again.

THOMAS MERTON

Whatever present challenges you face, remember what you have already successfully faced and come through. It's amazing, isn't it? Bring your courage and determination back to mind, feel it in your bones. You are more capable than you think.

To begin a new healthy habit, use the "When I, Then I" technique. Identify a specific thing you already do regularly, such as clean your teeth or get into bed, and add the new habit to this activity. For example, "When I clean my teeth, then I will think of three things I am grateful for." The existing activity is a solid base onto which you can build a new, constructive habit.

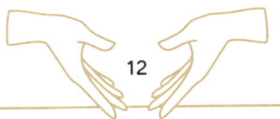

Don't start your day with the broken pieces of yesterday. Every day is a fresh start.

ANONYMOUS

Create a playlist of your favourite songs that helps you to relax, and a different playlist that lifts your energy levels and makes you want to dance. Music is a powerful way to move your mood in the direction you want to go.

A journal exercise for today: identify what you would like to do more often, and less often. Look at both lists and consider how you will shift things in your favour. This will strengthen your sense of agency in your life.

••• (15) •••

Gratitude is a powerful source of self-care. Research shows that practising gratitude each day improves optimism, heart health and your immune system. Notice what is going well for you and the people you care about.

Expand your ways of saying "no". Having boundaries that protect your time, resources and emotions is important and by no means negative in all situations. Experiment with these phrases: "Thanks, but not this time"; "What I need is something different"; "Not today, thank you."

Self-care doesn't mean that perfection is possible, where your well-being is in balance forever. In reality, self-care can be a progression towards recovering an inch of ground for yourself after a day when your family, colleagues or strangers have worn you out. Sometimes self-care is self-protection.

Check whether your caffeine intake is affecting your sleep quality. Caffeine is a stimulant and it suppresses the effects of adenosine (the chemical that builds up in the blood and makes you feel sleepy). It's best to avoid all caffeine products in the eight hours before bedtime. Remember that caffeine is found not only in coffee and tea but also in many energy drinks, soft drinks, chocolate and some painkillers.

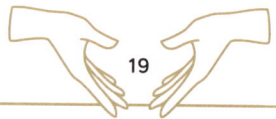

Restore your attention by dramatically slowing down whatever you're doing.

SHARON SALZBERG

Tonight, do something that helps your brainwaves move from an active beta state (analyzing and problem-solving) to alpha brainwaves (contemplating and daydreaming), which are associated with transitioning into a sleep-ready state. Examples include meditation, listening to relaxing music or reading.

Be curious about the things you tend to complain about the most. Everyone has something that gets on their nerves! What is it about this thing that really gets to you? Often there is a fear, worry or anger behind the complaining, such as not feeling safe enough, understood or respected. Bringing awareness to what you really need can empower you to act rather than feel helpless.

Bullet journalling is a way of monitoring what matters to you, helping with productivity and achieving goals. Whether listing events you are looking forward to, keeping your favourite affirmations in one place or tracking specific habits, give it a go.

Find time to be alone, away from the constant cycle of negative news. This might involve stepping outdoors or travelling somewhere. Solitude can be an opportunity to detox from the demands of others, helping you to feel more resilient.

Clean the mirrors and windows of your home. Just do one room if that is all you can manage. Notice what state they are in before you start, then feel the satisfaction as you clean them.

**Until you value yourself,
you won't value your time.
Until you value your time, you
will not do anything with it.**

M. SCOTT PECK

Write a list of what is on your mind. Next to each item, write whether you can take a positive action (or not). Prioritize these actions in order, focusing on those that are easiest and most realistic. Just recognizing what is on your mind by writing it down can help your brain to work on ideas and solutions while doing a task, during exercise or while you sleep.

The Swedish self-care concept of *lagom* (pronounced "*law-gum*") translates as "not too little, not too much". This approach invites you to live in a more balanced way. In which areas of your life is "not too little, not too much" already evident?

Find something outdoors that you think is beautiful: a leaf, an insect, a flower, a beautifully spun cobweb. Give it your attention. Notice the details. Reconnecting with the natural world reminds you that you are an expression of nature too.

Focus on doing one thing and complete it. Focusing on one thing reduces the scattering effect on your attention. You are less likely to make a mistake or miss an important detail, and you will feel more satisfaction as a result.

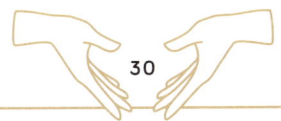

30

Instead of being like, "Oh my god, I'm so busy and stressed", I should be more like, "Oh, it's a good thing that I'm busy."

GK BARRY

31

Soften your expectations about sleeping well every night. If you do wake in the night, be careful to not fall into negative thoughts, such as *I should be able to sleep better* or *It shouldn't be like this.* Stress-related thoughts make it harder to sleep, triggering imaginary negative outcomes, so be kind to your mind.

april

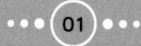

If you experience anxiety, acknowledge it – because fighting anxious thoughts or squashing anxious feelings only makes them stronger. Anxiety is a natural and necessary emotion. Ask yourself "What is the worst that can happen? What would I do then? How likely is the worst-case scenario?" Facing anxious thoughts helps them to be heard, processed and understood, giving you a way towards peace.

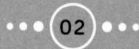

Clean your fridge to make sure it is hygienic. Remove the food contents carefully and clear out any products past their expiry date. Wipe clean the fridge shelves and any compartments, including in the door, before refilling with your produce. Practical actions like this are a reminder of what is in your control with self care.

Do the next and most necessary thing.

CARL JUNG

Journalling doesn't have to mean writing pages about your thoughts and feelings. Instead, write one sentence each day focusing on a single positive. What went well and why? Keeping track of one good thing each day soon accumulates, helping you to build a positive picture of yourself.

Your body is not a separate "thing" to you. Wherever you go, your body will be there too. What you do for your body you are doing for you. Check in today with how your body is feeling and consider what you can do to help it along, if necessary.

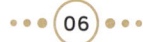

Lighten up on yourself. No one is perfect. Gently accept your humanness.

DEBORAH DAY

New questions generate new possibilities, so coach yourself using Sir John Whitmore's GROW model to guide you:

- Goal: What's your goal? Describe what it looks and sounds like.

- Reality: What are you already doing to achieve it? What's working? What isn't?

- Options: What else could you do? Make a list. Ask others for ideas.

- Will: What will you do and when? Take action and notice what happens.

And now that you don't have to be perfect, you can be good.

JOHN STEINBECK

Acknowledging loss – such as the loss of full health, a friendship or a work opportunity – can help you recognize what has happened and move on. Ways to openly acknowledge a loss include talking about it with a friend or noting it in a private journal.

Self-care means finding or creating a space where you can just be who you are without fear of judgement, whether from others or yourself. What do you notice when you let go of self-criticism and stop giving yourself a hard time about something?

Avoid the word "should" for the day. Why not, at least for today, swap "should" for "could"? What could you do for yourself today?

Grow herbs in your kitchen to bring some of the outdoors indoors. The vivid green shades and distinct aromas offer an enlivening sensory encounter right at your fingertips. Basil, coriander and chives are all easy to grow and will add exciting flavours to your food.

You are allowed to feel whatever you are feeling. You might understand why you feel upset, excited, angry or worried – or you might not. Acknowledging your feelings, whether with words, a doodle or a gesture, brings it to the surface, helping you deal with reality as it is.

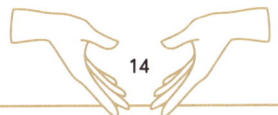

14

Keep good company, read good books, love good things and cultivate soul and body as faithfully as you can.

LOUISA MAY ALCOTT

Do you have a good book on the go or a regular magazine or newspaper you like to devour? Have you checked out new releases or revisited classics from the past? Reading enriches your world with new characters, vocabulary, ideas and stories, and has a calming effect on the mind.

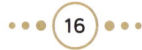

Who can you go for a walk and talk with? Sometimes it is easier to talk freely while your body is moving and the scenery is changing. The rhythm of walking, thinking and talking seems to work well together, offering physical and emotional benefits.

Don't be pressured into buying anything you don't truly want. Make sure you feel in control of what you buy, when and from whom, to avoid feeling regret later. It's true, the best things in life are free.

Express your anger safely without acting it out. Anger and self-care are not opposites but rather two sides of the same coin. Anger reveals who and what matters to you. Use words to express how you feel and why, not aggressive actions.

Studies show that the human heart detects and sends electromagnetic waves as part of the way we sense whether we are in tune with others around us. The heart understands some things before the rational brain. Listening to your heart is a pathway to wisdom and well-being.

Self-care means understanding your own value. Try this: write the words "I am…" at the top of a sheet of paper and list what comes to mind about who you are, including your roles (e.g. "I am a parent"), attributes (e.g. "I am resilient") and identities (e.g. your ethnicity, faith or purpose). Look down the list. What stands out to you?

A face mask is a great way to cleanse your skin, unclogging pores and leaving you feeling fresh. It can be good fun too and a chance for some funny photos. When else do you have the excuse to place cucumber slices over your eyes?

In what tone do you speak to yourself? Is it a gentle, caring tone, or is it more abrasive and critical? The "inner critic" can be relentless and impossible to please! Speak to it directly: "I hear you. Thank you for wanting to protect me."

•••(23)•••

What item can you safely repair today? Is there a piece of clothing or gadget that needs attention? Fixing things rather than throwing them away can save money and is better for the environment, increasing your sense of satisfaction.

Eating breakfast improves concentration by raising blood sugar levels and giving the brain a steady supply of glucose. Smelling food you enjoy increases dopamine levels and stimulates appetite – so don't miss out!

Self-care basics: Are you feeding your gut with healthy bacteria by eating a range of plant foods which match the different colours of the rainbow? Examples include: bananas, mangoes, red peppers, blueberries, leeks, grapes, sweet potatoes, figs, plums.

To love oneself is the beginning of a lifelong romance.

OSCAR WILDE

Courage comes before confidence. Is there something you have been wondering about learning, doing or saying? What will happen if you never take the risk? What could happen if you do? Live in the realm of positive probabilities rather than negative possibilities.

Reduce the amount of bright light you're exposed to in the evening to improve sleep. Turn down the brightness on the phones or gadgets you use. Dim room lights wherever possible and use lower-energy lightbulbs in lamps rather than using main lights. Reducing light exposure promotes the release of melatonin in the brain, helping you to feel sleepy and ready to rest.

Help the butterflies and bees by planting nectar-rich plants in your garden or in a community space (with permission). Their populations are in decline, which is a threat to their own existence and has an impact on human health too. Caring for the environment can give you a sense of accomplishment and a connection with something larger than yourself.

There is no such thing as "being normal". So, is there something you can laugh at yourself about? Not in a cruel way, just something you know is a bit ridiculous or a peculiar tendency you have. Self-care doesn't have to be all serious, so lighten up. Be like a feather!

may

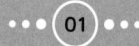

What is a challenge for you right now? Draw it on a piece of paper and colour it in. What does your challenge look like? Turning something that is invisible in your mind into a visible sketch can open up your thinking in a different way and offer solutions. Be curious about what your picture shows you.

Save money towards a treat or reward for yourself. Having something in mind, such as a music festival, a special new item of clothing or a meal out with friends, and gradually saving towards it, increases the sense of anticipation in the lead-up and, ultimately, the satisfaction when you reach your goal.

A journal exercise for today: list happy moments from your life going as far back as you choose. Write each down in a few words. Gather them together, all these glorious gifts that touched your heart and remain alive within you today. Feeling content and grateful is good for everything in your life.

Sometimes saying "no" to someone is necessary for you to say "yes" to yourself. Can you think of something you want to say "no" to but (perhaps secretly) feel you should say "yes" out of habit or fear of the other person's response? Stop keeping other people happy at a cost to your well-being.

Consider three ways you already practise self-care and name them. Why do they matter to you and how do they benefit you? Remind yourself, you are on this journey already.

Close your eyes and feel the air against your skin, perhaps on your face or your hands. Notice the gentleness of this contact. Doing this regularly during the day is a way of waking up again to the subtle flow of energy, a reminder that you are not separate from the world.

Tidy a corner of your home today so it looks and feels better to you (or just rearrange things and pretend it's tidier!). This is about doing something small where you notice an immediate difference with little effort.

**Knowing how to be solitary
is central to the art of loving.
When we can be alone, we can
be with others without using
them as a means of escape.**

BELL HOOKS

Reset after a difficult moment (as best as you can). Life is always unfolding in unexpected ways, so don't place too much meaning on something difficult. You already know that good things can come from difficult experiences. Go for a walk. Say to yourself, "Okay, let's go again." Every moment is new.

Grow something you can nurture; this could be a herb, flower or houseplant. Finding tangible ways to connect with your environment and look after something requiring regular care is a good discipline.

If you tend to get caught up in thoughts about the past or fantasizing about the future, notice how this intensifies your feelings. Exhale once forcefully out your mouth, as if blowing the thoughts away from your body. Come back to the here and now and you will feel stronger.

Switch off autopilot and do something different! Novelty can feel exciting and renew your sense about what's possible. Could you bake something new, watch an unusual show, go stargazing or play a new game with friends?

13

Self-love has very little to do with
how you feel about your outer self.
It's about accepting all of yourself.

TYRA BANKS

14

Reclaim using the words "I need…" There is nothing
needy or weak about identifying and stating what
you need. You might need practical assistance
with a task, information to make a decision or
simply to express your opinion. Hear yourself say
"What I need is…" out loud. Other people can't read
your mind, so how will they know unless you say?
Feeling understood activates natural opioids in the
body, helping with feelings of care and friendship.

Refresh the photographs you have in your home for an immediate visual impact. You don't have to throw the previous ones away. A small change can enliven your environment and remind you of the people you love and who love you.

Acknowledge thoughts about failure – *Yes, it is possible I might fail* – but then disobey those thoughts – *But I will attempt it anyway, do my best and see what happens*. This softens the power that thoughts about failing can have over you.

Follow a nudge. Perhaps you sense it is time to contact someone, read something or visit a certain place. Follow the nudge without knowing exactly why and discover what happens as a result. Listen to your intuition and it might lead to a good place.

Join a group or take up a voluntary role that fits with your lifestyle and which provides you with the opportunity to meet new people, for example, helping with an outdoors project or community initiative from time to time. Developing new social connections will enrich your learning and reduce feelings of isolation.

Reduce your need for everything to look just right and work out as planned without room for error. Not everyone has perfectionist tendencies, but they are common. Valuing excellence is a noble aim, but perfectionism causes strain. Instead, sometimes aim for "good enough" and learn from what works out differently to what you expected.

Don't be afraid to disagree. If you are not feeling heard or being taken seriously, then disagree in an agreeable way. Phrases such as "I hear your opinion and I have a different perspective..." can create a more truthful conversation benefitting everyone involved. Self-care means allowing yourself to be heard.

When you are travelling as a passenger, in a train, bus or car, look out of the window and let your mind wander, as if releasing a balloon into the sky. Daydreaming can be a safety valve for a busy mind, allowing unexpected insights to arise.

And here you are living despite it all.

RUPI KAUR

••• (23) •••

Offer genuine words of gratitude to others you meet today. It can be for simple things – the person who delivers your post or serves you in a shop. Notice how you feel when you express appreciation to others. Being a decent human costs nothing and will lift your spirits.

••• (24) •••

Don't work in bed. Keep the place where you sleep and the place where you work separate, especially if you work from home. Otherwise, the risk is that your mind will associate your bed with a state of alertness and, possibly, stress. Just like you (hopefully!) don't eat in the bathroom, keep good mental hygiene by physically separating sleep and work.

Placing a mirror behind indoor houseplants, such as in a bathroom, can increase the amount of light in a room as well as the visual perception of green – so it looks like there are more plants than there are. Seeing healthy plants has been shown to reduce stress hormones and improve memory. This can also be a way of saving money on plants!

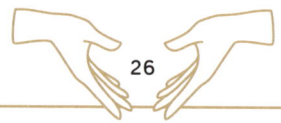

It takes courage to get out of bed in the morning and climb into the day.

EDWARD HIRSCH

Arrive early somewhere this week. Put your phone away, turn your face to the sky and bask in just being here, being you. You have come so far; why not notice this for yourself rather than chasing whatever is next?

Have a glass of water with your evening meal. Drinking water when you eat aids good digestion, maximizing the absorption of all the nutrients in your food.

••• 29 •••

Watch the sunset from a place where you can see as much of it as possible. Resist the urge to take photos, as this distances you from the immediate experience. Absorb the moments as the sun slips beneath the horizon, appreciating the changing colours and movement.

Be good to your skin. You'll wear it every day for the rest of your life.

RENÉE ROULEAU

Self-soothing is a way to calm the body and lower stress hormones. Place each hand on the opposite shoulder, as if you are hugging yourself. Slowly, but firmly, stroke down each arm with your hands, all the way to your fingertips. Allow your breathing to slow naturally. This activates the parasympathetic nervous system, helping the body to feel rested and safe.

june

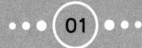

A golden rule of self-care is that it involves subtraction, not just addition. This might mean stopping a bad habit, unsubscribing from something, discarding items or removing yourself from a social group that doesn't feel healthy for you. What can you eliminate from your life today that will give you more of what you value?

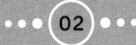

Download a meditation app and experiment with it. Lots of good-quality free apps are available (some require a small subscription). Apps provide regular reminders to practise, introduce you to new visualizations and provide added motivation. After all, talking about meditation isn't meditation. Meditation is meditation.

Going phone-free for a period of time that is a little outside your comfort zone, whether for an hour or a weekend, might be difficult if you are used to checking your phone constantly throughout the day. But doing so can improve your sleep and reduce your exposure to negative social comparisons.

First things first. Jot down what needs to be done and the first step for each. Start with the easiest and continue from there, just doing the next necessary thing. Breaking tasks into smaller steps engages parts of the brain that help with focus, memory and learning.

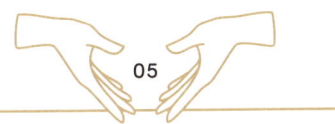

05

Do your little bit of good where you are; it's those little bits of good put together that overwhelm the world.

DESMOND TUTU

06

Remind yourself of what you are proud of, who you have helped, causes you have supported, opportunities you have created. Gather these truths together, however tiny or ordinary they seem, and notice the good you bring to the world. The world is a better place because you are in it.

••• 07 •••

A journal exercise for today: list the voices you choose to no longer listen to. Be it people from your past, sources in the media or negative chat you say to yourself. Turn down the volume on them and increase your inner peace.

••• 08 •••

Pamper yourself a little by massaging your hands with a hand cream after washing them to prevent your skin and cuticles becoming dry and itchy. Creams with sunflower-seed oil can help increase moisture levels.

••• 09 •••

Write a letter to a fictional or fantasy character. Tap into your desires and tell them what you really want! Perhaps this sounds ridiculous, but wishing can be a starting point for figuring out what you want and has been shown to boost mood.

When life is busy it is easy to forget the basics. Using visual reminders can help you sustain healthy hydration and dietary choices. Leaving a glass by the sink or a water bottle in a prominent place can help you stay hydrated. Keeping images of healthy foods or nutritious recipes in the kitchen can remind you to make positive food choices.

Rejuvenation means to gain fresh energy and happens through involvement with certain people, practices and places rather than with those that drain you. When you hear the word "rejuvenation" who, what and where comes to mind? Create space in your week for rejuvenation because you will think, feel and be a better person for it.

Adopt the pace of nature. Her secret is patience.

RALPH WALDO EMERSON

The ancient Buddhist practice of Tonglen involves breathing in the suffering of others (visualizing it as dark smoke) then breathing out peace, healing and harmony (visualizing your breath as warm, bright light). This practice helps you relate to your own suffering with gentleness and develop compassion towards others.

Don't compare the ways in which you care for yourself with what others do. If someone does something that inspires you, then adapt it for yourself. Do self-care your own way.

What is your favourite shape? Is it a circle, star, spiral, squiggle or something else? What is it about this shape that you like? Consider how the shape relates to your life story and let your mind wander about the shape of your life so far. Do these connections suggest any positive links or indicate any changes?

Keep your favourite fruits on hand. Fresh fruit is not only packed with vitamins, which are good for digestion and preventing colds, but it can also be a fun eating experience – peeling, squeezing, squashing, slicing! (Remember, in hot weather, most fruits should be kept in the fridge to help them last longer, except bananas!)

Self-care can involve shaking things up. Thirty seconds of cold water at the start of your shower activates your body's circulation and releases endorphins that reduce low moods. Tell yourself to "Be brave!" as you stand under the freezing water.

You are not superhuman, so remember to ask for help when you need it – whether it is for a practical task or for emotional support in a situation. Help is like breathing; it is something that needs to both flow in and out. Self-care is not always a solitary process.

Send a text or call a friend who has been on your mind. Reaching out to someone can be reassuring and motivating. Who knows what you will talk about given the chance.

Electrolytes, such as sodium, potassium and magnesium, are chemicals that conduct electricity when dissolved in water, helping to regulate nerve and muscle function and repairing damaged muscle tissue. Adding a thin slice of lemon or cucumber to a glass of water will enrich your body with electrolytes.

Making things with your hands can be incredibly satisfying. Whether it is with food or craft materials, in the garden or in the garage, creative activity can reduce stress. Losing yourself in an activity like this can be replenishing for both the mind and body, and you will have something to show for your efforts.

Give and receive hugs. Safe physical touch, whether hugs, holding hands or a massage, is good for releasing oxytocin (the brain chemical associated with feelings of connection), lowering stress and anxiety. Safe touch connects you with others. Cuddling a pet has the same benefits.

Rather than something to be afraid of, silence is a rare gift and has its own voice. You don't have to talk to yourself all the time, trying to figure things out. Silence opens the door for stillness and new strength.

A good pedicure is a chance to refresh your feet and take care of your cuticles and nails. Whether you arrange for someone to do this for you or you do it yourself, your feet will be grateful.

What positive stories in the news, whether local or international, are inspiring you? Every day, wherever you look, there will be people helping others, showing care and creating hope. These moments might get lost among the news headlines highlighting suffering, but look out for what is good, including from dedicated websites that promote good news, and let yourself be inspired.

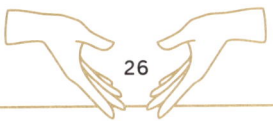

The most important decision you make is to be in a good mood.

VOLTAIRE

Stretch! Go on to your tiptoes, point your arms towards the sky, inhale deeply, then slowly bring your arms down to your side and lower your heels to the ground. Slow, deliberate stretching of your muscles for a few minutes a day improves the suppleness of your body and lifts your mood.

Be a self-care advocate with men you know. Many men feel pressured to "act strong" and "have it together", causing them to hide their true feelings and deny real problems. Use your voice to challenge damaging stereotypes because helping others in this way will help you to experience your own courage and strength.

Goals are good for setting a direction, but systems are best for making progress.

JAMES CLEAR

Try to stop worrying because it steals your joy. One way to do this, because it is easier to say than do, is to catch yourself when worrying thoughts occur and say "Stop!" out loud. This is not about criticizing yourself but rather protecting yourself in the same way you would say "Stop!" to a child if they were about to hurt themselves. This can empower you to have more control over your thought processes.

july

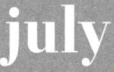

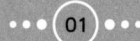

Optimism is a muscle you have to exercise. People who choose an optimistic perspective tend to be physically healthier, have a better diet and live longer. Optimism also lowers levels of fibrinogen in the liver, which is responsible for blood clots. Consider a situation and ask yourself "What good things are possible?"

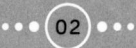

Lifting weights can improve your balance, muscle mass and bone density. This releases the brain chemical dopamine, which gives you the feeling of motivation. Light dumbbells for your biceps are a good place to start, but don't strain or do too much in one go. A few minutes on a daily basis is better than overdoing it.

Understanding others better requires openness and curiosity. For example, rather than blaming someone for something, assume they have good intentions and explore how the situation could work out better. Seeking to understand others strengthens your mental agility.

If you have the ability to love, love yourself first.

CHARLES BUKOWSKI

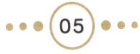

If the door of your refrigerator is covered in magnets, photos and pieces of paper, then why not play around with a new design? Remove old items and add new photos, drawings, puzzles or magnets. Have fun being a fridge artist.

Cancel something non-essential and give yourself a night off. Maybe you want to save some money, have a quiet night in or just take some time for yourself. Allowing yourself to choose is a vital self-care tactic.

Go for a lunchtime walk. However busy you are, prioritize walking outdoors for at least 15–20 minutes. The combination of fresh air, movement and changing your sensory experience can increase your energy for the rest of the day.

Take short breaks to increase your focus and ability to work in a sustainable way. A break is not just a caffeine top-up but also a genuine pause.

Help your bedding smell extra fresh by adding half a cup of baking soda to your usual laundry detergent. Wash on a temperature of 40–60°C (100–140°F). Neutralizing bad odours can make your environment more comfortable and relaxing.

Learn about a specific self-care theme you are interested in. Find an inspiring video or podcast related to this topic and immerse yourself in it. Afterwards, ask yourself what you will do differently in light of what you have learned.

Check your consumption of diuretics: drinks that make you need the toilet more often, such as those containing caffeine and alcohol. Notice when you naturally feel thirsty and balance your hydration with fresh water to prevent headaches and fatigue.

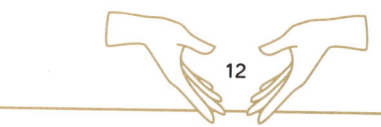

12

We do not remember days.
We remember moments.

CESARE PAVESE

Go fruit picking – whatever is in season where you are – and use what you pick to make something delicious. Whether it is fruit smoothies, a fruit salad, crumble, jam or a pie, there will be such satisfaction in knowing that you hand-picked what you are eating. If it turns out well, why not share it with others?

Self-care is a priority
and we have to do it more.

AVA DuVERNAY

Listen to your body. If you're thirsty, drink plenty
of water, if you're hungry, enjoy a healthy snack, if
you need to move your body, engage in an exercise
that you enjoy.

Make it easier to snack on healthier foods and
harder to eat junk. Place nuts, dried fruit and
seeds (depending on your taste preferences) in a
bowl and have them within reach of your desk or
near the kettle. Move the cookie jar out of view and
hide processed foods behind other items.

If you have made a mistake you feel guilty about, acknowledge your feeling but don't indulge in feeling bad. If there is something to learn or a way to make amends, then do so. Treating yourself with compassion is far better for your sleep, concentration and productivity than hanging onto guilt.

Rest your eyes from digital devices. Long periods of staring at a screen can cause headaches and hurt your eyes. Every 20 minutes give your eyes a 20-second rest and look at something 20 steps away, perhaps out of a window. If you wear glasses or contact lenses, remove them and squeeze your eyes shut and open again to restore the tear film and lubricate your eyes.

19

Try not to take yourself too seriously. Life isn't always easy, but it is easier when you stop trying so hard to impress other people. Honestly, you are doing fine just being the person you already are. Remember, smiling releases naturally occurring chemicals that elevate your mood.

20

The challenge is not to be perfect – it is to be whole.

JANE FONDA

21

Check in with how your body is feeling so you can provide what it needs. How are your energy levels? If you are feeling run down, consider eating more fresh fruit, taking a vitamin C supplement and going to bed earlier to accelerate your recovery.

Drinking tea in the morning is hydrating (unlike coffee) and helps with blood circulation. Black tea and green tea can lower blood sugar levels and are full of flavonoids, which support good heart health. Health experts recommend no more than four cups of tea a day.

The body can accumulate tension throughout the day, so use this exercise to release it: squeeze both of your hands into fists and at the same time breathe in through your nose. Count to three and hold this position. Then, breathing out through your mouth, open both hands at the same time, spreading your fingers apart. Repeat three times: squeeze then release. Notice the contrast.

Playing with pets can be wonderful for lifting your mood and taking your mind off other matters. Animals don't judge you. Research shows that playing with dogs increases the hormones that elevate good feelings.

Self-care is not "just another thing to do". You probably do more than you realize but might not label it as "self-care". For some people, self-care might mean repairing the car, weeding the garden or going to a comedy show. If it helps your body, mind and soul, then it's self-care.

Even if it makes others uncomfortable, I will love who I am.

JANELLE MONÁE

Take a photo of a messy area of your home, then devote 10 minutes to cleaning it. Set a timer and race against the clock to see how much you can get cleaned in the time. Choosing a "finish time" can make the task feel more manageable. Compare the "before" and "after" images for a feeling of satisfaction.

Get yourself a teapot with a design that makes you smile. Maybe it reminds you of someone or somewhere you love. Each time you use it, that connection will be present. If drinking tea isn't your thing, then consider what you could buy for yourself that will connect you with special moments, people and places you cherish.

Ruminating thoughts and being "in your own head" too much could indicate excessive activity in the default mode network in the brain. Ways to reset this include walking in nature, mindfulness exercises and deep breathing, which promote a more calm, focused state of mind.

He hauora te taonga.
(Health is wealth.)

MĀORI PROVERB

Whenever possible, welcome your experience without reacting to it. Accepting the come-and-go of your experience without judging it or trying to change it can bring you more serenity and perspective.

august

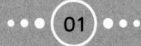

Establish a bedtime and stick to it. Regularly getting more than 7 hours of sleep a night will ensure you feel rested and decrease the risk of you being unwell. Your body's natural sleep rhythms work best with predictability, so set yourself a reminder.

Turn down the volume on catastrophizing and increase your calm. If you tend to think that things will go wrong, try to recognize that your mind is overdoing it. Challenge yourself – are those negative things likely to happen? What is more realistic? Remember you have strengths to draw on too.

Self-care might mean campaigning on an issue that matters to you. Think of people you know who share your values. What does positive, collective action look like? Be heard, take action and feel positive.

Create a daily "Yay!" list. Maybe you unexpectedly found something you thought was lost, received a surprise message from a friend or enjoyed a song on the radio. A "Yay!" list helps you recognize pleasant things in life.

Play! Maybe this sounds childish, but adults need playtime too. Studies show that playfulness encourages creativity, stimulates good feelings, creates connections with others and reduces levels of stress. What does playing more look like to you?

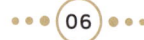

When was the last time you danced? Everyone dances differently and whether it is fast or slow, on your own or with others, dancing can improve your heart health and physical co-ordination as well as release feelings of joy. Go on, have a dance!

Don't judge your day too soon just because it doesn't start well. A difficult hour doesn't have to equal a bad day or a bad life. Try to refrain from prematurely judging anything because things often work out well later on.

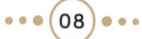

Unsubscribe from advertising and updates you don't read, need or enjoy. You won't miss out on anything important and you might appreciate fewer interruptions and less unnecessary noise in your life.

09

A mantra is a short, positive saying that gets you into the right mindset to start, continue or complete a task, for example, "Just do it" or "Back yourself". What mantra would you choose to face a present challenge?

10

Use a puzzle book to occupy your brain rather than your phone. Puzzles are ideal for filling short chunks of time, perhaps during a break or while waiting for someone. This will reduce the amount of on-screen stimuli that bombards your brain, promoting rest and creativity instead.

11

Give yourself a chance to roam. Roaming doesn't have to mean a long distance or on your own. Roam somewhere away from the concrete and traffic and enjoy a different view.

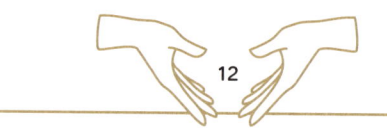

12

Nourishing yourself in a way that helps you blossom in the direction you want to go is attainable, and you are worth the effort.

DEBORAH DAY

Sleep is the foundation of good self-care. Good sleepers don't have complicated strategies but instead create the conditions where good sleep is more likely. Having at least an hour away from screens and visual stimuli before bedtime helps. Enjoying a few minutes of breathing out long, slow breaths also releases stress – and can get you yawning!

The boundary lines between home and work can become blurred. To help retain the balance, have a mindful moment before you start your work or a lunchtime stroll without checking emails. A balanced approach will improve the quality of your work and your well-being.

Research shows that an active social life protects against memory loss and anxiety. Is there a great pub, cafe or park where you enjoy hanging out with friends? Take the lead and make it happen.

You are the expert on you. There will always be plenty of advice about how you can improve your life. The intention is to help, but you know yourself best, so remember to do what works for you.

I don't have any time to stay up all night worrying about what someone who doesn't love me has to say about me.

VIOLA DAVIS

Having a constellation of support where you can talk openly with others you trust is vital for self-care. If there are more private matters you want to talk through, your friends might not be sufficiently independent or suitably qualified. Consider speaking with a trained therapist, whether one to one or in a small confidential group.

Try something for the first time to activate your curiosity. Learn the basics of another language, join a writing group or make a meal you have never attempted before. Become a beginner and enjoy the learning process rather than the result.

Around 20–30 per cent of the fluid you need each day to keep hydrated comes from the food you eat. Tomatoes, apples, peaches, melon, courgettes, celery, broccoli and cucumber all have high water content and contribute towards your hydration, preventing fatigue and headaches.

There's an old saying: "Take time to smell the roses." Take this wise advice on board. Lean in, close your eyes, breathe in the scent of something pleasant and feel enlivened.

Creative writing is a way to slow down, untangle your thoughts and gain insight into yourself. Find an ordinary object that interests you and become curious about it. Imagine the story of where it came from or write something from its perspective, as if the object can think, feel and speak. If this object had a message for you, what would it be?

Depending on your dairy tolerance and taste preferences, consider plant-based milk alternatives in your diet, such as almond or oat milk. Oat milk is a high-fibre option with vitamin B for energy, and almond milk is rich in vitamin E, which supports the immune system. Look for "No added sugar" options.

Live simply so others can simply live.

MAHATMA GANDHI

After exercising, it is important to consume antioxidants to neutralize the damage done by free radicals (unstable atoms that cause illness and ageing). Foods and fluids that are beneficial are those containing b-carotene and vitamins C and E, such as bananas, blueberries, tomatoes, strawberries and dark chocolate.

Every day you are exposed to toxins, whether in the environment or in additives in processed foods or from emotional stress. Drinking fresh water flushes out harmful toxins, cleansing the body and supporting better well-being.

Be brave and disconnect from anyone or anything on social media that doesn't add value to your life. If any content makes you feel worth "less" – stop engaging with it immediately.

It's not selfish to love yourself, take care of yourself, and make your happiness a priority. It's necessary.

MANDY HALE

••• 29 •••

Rest your hands gently over your heart then ask yourself a question you want an answer to. Let your heart speak, perhaps through an image or phrase that comes to mind. Your heart knows things your head will never understand.

••• 30 •••

If you feel upset or angry about something, go for a walk outside (somewhere safe). Rather than rehearsing angry thoughts as you walk, breathe in deeply as you move, stamp your feet on the ground, clench your fists and release them. These small actions can soften the intensity of the initial emotion, helping you to think more clearly and move towards peace.

••• 31 •••

Practising self-care has multi-faceted benefits. For example, going to a music show with a friend can be great for your mood as well as your friendship, and afterwards you might have photographs to cherish the memory. This crossover shouldn't be a surprise because you are a whole person, not merely a set of categories: physical, mental, social, etc.

september

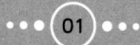

Self-care isn't the latest trend but has its origins in ancient practices (such as mindfulness meditation) and is evident in diverse cultures across the world, especially in the Nordic countries and South-East Asia. Learn about self-care from a culture or part of the globe you are less familiar with and expand the ways you can enhance your well-being.

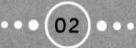

Why not explore an app to support a particular aspect of your self-care? Some apps can track your nutrition habits and generate suggestions for healthy eating, and others can recommend breathing exercises to aid in calming you down when you feel stressed. (Technology cannot replace the advice of a medical professional or counsellor where needed.)

I'm either going to love me or hate me. And I chose to love myself.

QUEEN LATIFAH

Be mindful when completing an ordinary task. Take a breath. Appreciate the value of what you have done for yourself (and possibly others). Noticing the ordinary activities of your day is a way of feeling present and more alive.

Exfoliate dry or chapped skin with a homemade sugar scrub. Mix together 85 g (3 oz) of sugar with two tablespoons (1 fl oz) of vegetable oil. You can add some essential oils, such as lavender, peppermint or tea tree oil. Dampen your skin and rub on the scrub, then rinse with tap water.

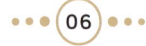

Check your diet for how much you are consuming from each of these categories:

- "Go" foods (carbohydrates that fuel the body, such as bread, oats, pasta, rice and potatoes)
- "Grow" foods (proteins that repair the body, such as fish, cheese and meat)
- "Glow" foods (fruit and vegetables)

Balancing nutrients maintains your energy and boosts your well-being.

Research into sleep quality consistently indicates that an adult requires at least 7 hours each night so your body can restore and repair itself, healing tired muscles. When you turn out the light at night, focus on taking several deep breaths to activate your parasympathetic nervous system, helping your body to relax.

Gather together items that no longer bring you joy. Don't overthink it, just collect books, objects, clothes and whatever else you feel has had its time. Recycle or regift what you can. How does it feel to create more space, ready for something new?

It does not matter how slowly you go as long as you do not stop.

CONFUCIUS

There is no magic wand with which to restore good sleep, but mindfulness can assist. In bed, bring your attention to your senses. Taking deep breaths in and exhaling long breaths out through your mouth often help the body relax.

Whatever "doing nothing" means to you today (or one day soon), do that. Give yourself the opportunity to get lost in a good movie or book, chill out to your favourite music or ramble somewhere you choose with someone you love.

Consider which self-care practice you'd like to do more regularly. Use notifications and pleasant-sounding alarms to give yourself a regular nudge. At least then you will have a conscious choice to make, rather than forgetting by accident.

••• 13 •••

Check out local places that offer bargain-priced food and drinks to be collected at the end of the day. You might pick up a real treat that brightens your day while helping to cut food waste at the same time.

Foraging sustainably for wild fruits can be a fun adventure, connecting you with your environment and introducing you to new places. Edible fruits such as blackberries and wild raspberries are often found along canals. Check they are ripe before eating them and only forage from a bountiful source.

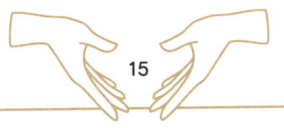

When you recover or discover something that nourishes your soul and brings joy, care enough about yourself to make room for it in your life.

JEAN SHINODA BOLEN

Take a "forest bath" (an ancient Japanese practice known as *shinrin yoku*), which has been shown to reduce stress hormones, lower blood pressure and generate feelings of happiness and ease. Immerse yourself in the experience of being among trees larger, stronger and older than you.

If you are having a terrible day, for whatever reason, even little things can add to your woes. What would provide you with a moment of refuge and lift your spirits? Perhaps a favourite food or song, or spending the day with a friend? Tomorrow is a new day where new things become possible.

Turn up the tunes! Listen, sing or dance along to a song you love as a way to reconnect with your own voice, body and power.

"Taste your food, not your troubles" is an old Zen proverb, a reminder to savour the moment. Remove distractions and immerse yourself fully in experiencing the aroma, taste and texture of your food. Eating mindfully improves digestion and cultivates thankfulness for what you have.

Accept yourself, love yourself, and keep moving forward.

ROY T. BENNETT

Reconnect with a previous tip in this book that has meaning for you. Self-care isn't about novelty and endless new ideas but practising what you know to be helpful, true and nurturing for yourself. Go ahead, flick through the book and remind yourself.

Rather than asking yourself "Why do I feel this way?", which will lead to self-analysis, ask yourself "From whom or where is this feeling coming from?" This question brings about an awareness of your relationships, past or present. Maybe the feeling is coming from within you or maybe it belongs to someone else. Care, but don't carry the emotions of others.

Enjoy the superpowers of tomatoes! Tomatoes are rich in vitamins A, B, C and E, boosting your immune system, improving gut health and keeping teeth, skin and bones healthy. Tomatoes help with male sperm motility, and the potassium in them lowers cholesterol. Tomatoes are easy to grow or find in local markets and shops.

Gardens offer a variety of ways to feel calm and gain a sense of accomplishment. Weeding, raking up leaves, pruning plants and harvesting vegetables help to burn calories and strengthen muscles, and being outdoors will increase your levels of vitamin D and calcium.

A journal exercise for today: what is your favourite season or time of year, and why? Appreciating the seasons can help you to calibrate your own rhythms in life.

Name your hobbies out loud. Hobbies are a brilliant way of relieving stress and unleashing your creativity and talent. What do you love pursuing in your own time? If you have let a hobby drift, take action and set yourself a date to take it up again.

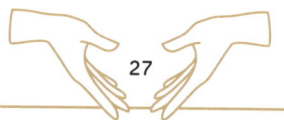

27

Treat yourself like someone you love.

GLENNON DOYLE

28

Explore the Japanese well-being concept of *ikigai* (pronounced *ee-key-guy*), a fusion of two words meaning "life" and "the realization of hope". *Ikigai* invites you to live a life that is meaningful by reflecting on what you love doing, what you are good at, what the world needs and what you can be paid for. Where these four aspects overlap – that's your *ikigai*!

Regular meditation has been shown to increase blood flow to an area of the brain called the anterior cingulate cortex, which plays a significant role in controlling thoughts, emotions and attention. Meditation doesn't have to be for hours at a time; even just ten minutes a day focusing on your breathing can help reduce anxiety.

Indulge your imagination by writing a poem, a story or a piece of music, or by making a drawing. Don't judge what you create, just unleash your feelings. Make it as ridiculous or as romantic as you want. Spontaneous creativity that expresses your truth (or fantasy) can help you and others see the world differently.

october

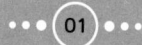

Do your best not to over-commit yourself. Even if you love making plans and being busy, everyone has limits, so check what is coming up in your diary and be realistic about what you say "yes" to. A full diary is not a sign of success if it costs you rest, family time or your sanity.

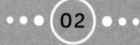

Be at the centre of your own world for a few moments. Shut the door. Unplug technology. Ignore emails. Step out of the whirlwind of the world and savour the present moment. Breathe in. Notice your shoulders rise a little as you inhale. You are here!

Lighting in a room can affect moods and energy levels. Dimming lights in your home environment helps promote melatonin, the brain chemical that helps you feel sleepy. Placing fairy lights and scented candles around a room can also create a warm ambience.

Make lists in a notes app or use apps that nudge you on hydration, track your sleep or provide positive daily affirmations. Make your tech enhance your well-being.

The most common way people give up their power is by thinking they don't have any.

ALICE WALKER

Every "body" is different, and every "body" changes as it ages. It is important to communicate what you need during times of reduced mobility (such as having an injury or illness) and significant transition (such as the perimenopause). Physical changes don't just affect the biological body but they can also impact emotional well-being, energy levels, sleep, memory and your sense of who you are. Consider what support you need.

Check your soaps. Many soaps today contain an ingredient called SLS (sodium laureth sulfate), a synthetic detergent that foams easily. However, it also strips skin of its natural oils and can clog pores and cause acne. If your skin tends to get itchy and dry, consider changing to SLS-free soaps.

••• 08 •••

What is a comforting bedtime ritual for you? It could include holding a hot (decaffeinated) drink, wrapping yourself in a blanket, sitting in a cosy place and watching something you find interesting. Comfort helps the body's central nervous system to settle.

••• 09 •••

Baking is a chance to slow down. Whether you bake flapjacks, fairy cakes, fresh bread or pizza, enjoy the aromas and textures of the ingredients. Why not involve friends, children or a partner? The baking experience is just as important as the result.

••• 10 •••

Do something different this week. Put aside your projects or studies and venture outdoors with someone you love. Get out of your head and back into your body to help ground yourself.

Self-care strengthens your autonomy when you need to make choices about what you create or tolerate in your life. If something or someone is a source of distress for you, don't ignore it. If this means taking a brave step today and asking for help, please do this for yourself.

Diffusing a few drops of essential oils into clean water in a diffuser can be relaxing and help to reduce anxiety and stress. Around six to eight drops is enough but add less if you have children around and make sure the room is well ventilated. Popular essential oils include rosemary, lavender, bergamot, yang ylang and geranium.

Self-care can mean taking a balanced approach to money. If you have a debt, are you reducing it? If you have credit cards, are you paying them off each month? If you have savings, what is your intention for them? Money is a wonderful servant and if you're in control, your stress levels will be lower.

Be disciplined, whether it is with exercise, participating in a club or completing a qualification. Metaphorically, you don't sow a seed in a garden one day only to dig it up the next day to check if it is growing. Tiny actions accumulate over time. Consider using a notebook, reminders or a relevant app to help you remain disciplined.

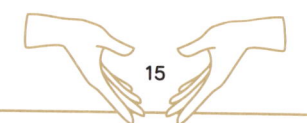

15

Do your thing and don't care if they like it.

TINA FEY

16

Confidence is a quality that, for many people, comes and goes. A shortcut to helping feelings of confidence return is to remember the times in your life when you felt confident. What did you see, hear and do? Relive these moments. How did it feel and what did the confidence give you? Nobody else on earth is the same as you so step forward with being you!

A journal exercise for today: make a "top ten" list. This could be songs, movies, cars or places to go. It can be fun to remember sources of enjoyment you have experienced and to play around with those you like the most and why.

Do your best to stop agonizing over setbacks beyond your control. Shift 100 per cent of your attention towards what is within your control, even if this is just your next breath, next sentence, next step. Moving forwards in this way generates hope.

••• 19 •••

Who says you need to know all the answers? To some extent, everyone is making up their lives as they go along. Caring for yourself during times of uncertainty is an anchor, not an escape. It is okay to say, "I don't know yet."

Ensure your time at work is used wisely by checking why you have been invited to a meeting or event. Perhaps you have other priorities and responsibilities the other person isn't aware of? Negotiate your involvement rather than attending out of habit and feeling resentful. Stay accountable to yourself for doing good work.

What rewards motivate you? Rewards help activate dopamine, the feel-good brain chemical, and move you to act towards a goal (or just something you want to do). Reward yourself at the end of the process. You're not too old to have a self-care sticker chart if that will serve you!

If you're not inspired by the word "exercise", think about "movement" instead. Going up and down stairs, vacuuming your home and walking the dog are all forms of movement that get your heart rate going and, so, improve your health. Sometimes just moving is the important thing.

The perfect self-care routine doesn't exist, so meet yourself where you are. Keep your approach realistic and doable and you will reap the benefits.

Setting a goal is useful for choosing a direction in life. This doesn't have to be a life-changing challenge – it might be a small goal that stirs you into action. Decide what you want to achieve and by when. Having goals can help you feel constructive and capable of action.

Be patient with yourself. Self-growth is tender; it's holy ground. There's no greater investment.

STEPHEN COVEY

Today, practise doing one thing at a time. Modern life can be full of rushing, meeting other people's demands and constant interruptions through technology. When you walk down the stairs, just walk down the stairs without rushing. When you make a hot drink, focus on the task. When in conversation, give your full attention to the person. This is a more centred way of living and will increase your sense of purpose and calm.

Give your toes a quick workout in the morning before getting out of bed. Curl and uncurl them several times. This exercise can help prevent a foot injury known as *plantar fasciitis*. Squeezing each toe with your fingers will improve blood circulation and reduce cramp.

Drinking water first thing in the morning replaces lost moisture from exhalation during the night. Even mild dehydration impairs your ability to think clearly. Drink a glass of water while waiting for the kettle to boil for your morning drink.

Run yourself a warm bath and drop a scented bath bomb into the water. Another option is to add bath salts to help relax muscles and ease joint pain, particularly beneficial after strenuous exercise or a busy day on your feet.

Maintaining personal hygiene through grooming yourself can be a way to de-stress and reconnect with yourself. Whether it is flossing between your teeth and gums, caring for your nails or moisturizing your skin, doing something that helps you to feel cleaner and fresher and look your best is wonderful self-care.

If other people live with you, ask for their observations on your self-care practice. What do they think you do well? (Perhaps you inspire them!) Is there something you are not doing as much as usual? Maybe there are things you do well that they could get your advice on, and vice versa. Teaming up can multiply the rewards.

november

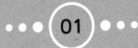

For sleeping, make sure your bedroom is as dark as possible (unless this is a phobia!). Remove sources of bright light, such as devices that have standby lights. Having thick curtains, wearing an eye mask and using a draught excluder to block light coming from beneath the bedroom door can all help darken your room and improve your chances of sleeping well.

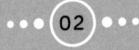

Healthy self-care includes giving to others that which you most desire. Who else can you celebrate today? Shift your focus for a moment and offer someone else sincere words of praise and recognition. Being generous is a gift to your own well-being.

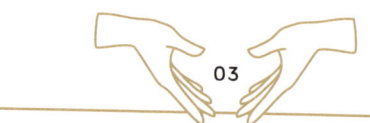

03

Almost everything will work again if you unplug it for a few minutes, including you.

ANNE LAMOTT

If your home suffers from damp walls during the winter months, this can affect your breathing, immune system and skin. Consider investing in a dehumidifier, which is effective in not only removing moisture from the air but also removing dust and musty odours. An additional benefit is that dehumidifiers help washed clothes dry more quickly. Caring for your environment is a way of caring for yourself.

Sleeping beneath a weighted blanket on your bed can improve sleep, as the weight can help the body to feel grounded and calm. (If you choose to try this, for safety purposes, always check the weights are suitable for the person's size and age.)

Self-care makes your use of time more sustainable.

JACK KORNFIELD

Sometimes self-care means having a challenging conversation. If you need to resolve something with someone, prepare yourself by being clear about what you would like the outcome to be. Seek to understand. Stay respectful. Listen as much as you speak. Difficult conversations are opportunities for mutual learning.

Moods are affected by many factors, including hormone changes during the month, genetics, the amount of time spent outdoors, daily hydration and diet, so don't let feeling low define your story. Tomorrow is a new day and another chance to take positive action.

If you're reading a book or watching a TV series that you're not enjoying, don't feel bad about letting it go. Give yourself the choice rather than abiding by an arbitrary obligation.

Try to practise self-restraint in an emotionally charged situation. Let things settle before you react. Remember, most situations unfold and move on without a need to stir them up into something they don't need to be.

If a small stress arises, practise "breathing with". This is when you observe an emotional discomfort you feel and gently bring your attention back to your breath while the discomfort is there. You are with it, not forcing it to change. Practising this during small difficulties may help when something more challenging arises.

Check whether you are consuming too many ultra-processed foods (UPFs), such as crisps, ham, biscuits, cereals, sausages or ready meals. The ingredients used in UPFs carry health risks and can potentially lead to Type 2 diabetes and obesity. Consider swapping them for fresh foods that are higher in fibre, minerals and vitamins. Remember, foods affect moods!

Breathe. Let go. And remind yourself that this very moment is the only one you know you have for sure.

OPRAH WINFREY

Give yourself a self-care gift. What would you truly love to receive? Perhaps it is a day walking along the coast, a fancy seasonal beverage, a new music album or a special hand cream. You don't have to tell anybody or justify the gift. It can be your secret.

Take a brisk walk outdoors to increase your exposure to daylight. What colours, scents, movement and sounds are present? Let the environment invigorate you.

Give yourself the best start and prepare for tomorrow, today. This might be making a lunch for yourself, choosing what you will wear and identifying your priorities for tomorrow. Planning ahead will give you confidence and boost your mood.

If you feel the need to cry, then go ahead. Of course, you can't force this and maybe now isn't quite the moment. Crying is not a sign of weakness; it restores the brain's ability to think clearly by flushing out stress hormones.

Excessive noise can affect hearing, heart rate, stress levels and sleep. Reduce the amount of unwelcome noise you experience by using noise-cancelling headphones during the day and earplugs at night.

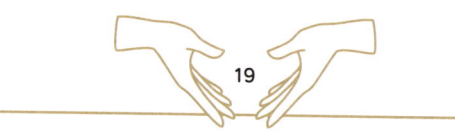

19

Loving yourself isn't an act of arrogance. It's an act of survival.

YARA SHAHIDI

Self-care isn't about getting top grades in every area of your life. Life is not school! Drop the idea of being a perfect parent, sibling, friend, partner, socialite and colleague. What area of your life could you let slide, at least for a bit, where you don't have to be 100 per cent on it? Less strain helps relationships flow more naturally and will reduce stress.

Ground yourself by pressing your heels into the spot where you're standing. Grounding has been shown to reduce stress, accelerate the healing of wounds and improve sleep.

Illuminate your day by having a bright lamp on by your bedside in the early mornings to stimulate feelings of wakefulness. Research indicates that 20 minutes of increased light exposure in the morning can help improve mood and concentration during the day.

Eat yourself well with food combinations that help the amino acid tryptophan increase the uptake of serotonin, which energizes the whole body, for example, salmon and brown rice, peanut butter on toast or a mix of seeds and nuts.

List the places where you feel able to replenish your energy. This might include a particular chair in a room at home, your garden, the gym or a favourite exercise route, a bench in a local park or a walk by a river. They don't have to be solitary or quiet places – there might be a cafe, group activity or sports venue that you enjoy visiting because it lifts your spirits. Let the diversity of the world revitalize you!

Return to self-care basics today: how is your personal hygiene? Are you getting sufficient time outdoors? Do you have people you trust to talk to? If you are feeling tired or low, any self-care action might feel impossible. Do what you can. This itself is heroic.

Adopt a growth mindset if something hasn't worked out for you. Identify three useful things from the experience and focus on these and what lessons they offer, because learning moves you forward.

You deserve respect, so don't accept mistreatment from anyone, especially if it questions your self-worth. Whether it is sarcastic comments or someone talking down to you, remember your needs are valid and you don't have to tolerate unkindness.

Talk to yourself like you would to someone you love.

BRENÉ BROWN

Embrace the less exciting bits of your day. When you daydream or have a rest, a group of brain regions called the default mode network becomes active, generating new insights and connections. Mundane activities like hanging out the washing or tidying up become perfect moments for insight to occur. Your brilliance is always available.

It is important to keep your body supple and reduce stiffness, especially in the colder months. Explore a practice like yoga, which offers simple ways to increase physical flexibility through static poses, or Pilates, which uses movement to tone muscles and strengthen your core. Looking after your body in this way will help with your sleep and moods.

december

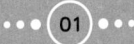

Different times of the year provide an opportunity for recognizing endings and beginnings in the cycle of life. Whether it's Diwali, Hanukkah, Yule, Christmas, Hogmanay or something else, festivals provide an opportunity to return to what has meaning for you, and to celebrate life through rituals and traditions, often with family and community. How do you like to celebrate these times? Celebrating can replenish your sense of joy, purpose and connection with others and nature.

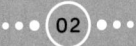

Consider your alcohol consumption for the week. Switching to low-alcohol or alcohol-free options could restore your hydration and regulate your sleep, as well as lowering your risk of illness. This can also be a way of saving money.

Self-care is how you take your power back.

LALAH DELIA

Introduce plants into your home that are good at absorbing moisture from the air; this could include ferns, peace lilies, orchids and aloe vera. These plants improve air quality and can reduce signs of damp, which can negatively affect breathing.

Take care of what you say to yourself because your body is listening. Name problematic thoughts, for example, "That's just an angry thought" or "That sounds like self-pity". You are not your thoughts. Naming thoughts out loud prevents them solidifying into a story you act out.

06

Refresh the contents of your fridge and cupboards. Consider whether the food and drink you buy reflects the values you aspire to, such as healthy produce, locally grown goods or products that have organic and ethical credentials. What you consume can have a positive effect on your hormones, body-chemistry and moods.

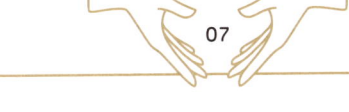

07

The most powerful relationship you will ever have is the relationship with yourself.

STEVE MARABOLI

Be careful if you get "mentally gripped" by someone or something that brings out the worst in you. The clues will be that your body and face tighten up, your tone of voice will change and you will feel you have less freedom in how to respond. Don't stay in this state of mind. Take a deep breath, be aware and release your tension.

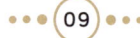

Remember your resilience by using these sentence starters:

- "I am..." – these are statements about your positive personal qualities.

- "I can..." – these are statements about your choices and capabilities.

- "I have..." – these are statements about your life experiences.

Keep them positive. Next time you face a challenge, remember who you are.

Achieve some winter comfort by keeping your feet cosy during cold weather. Heat rises, so wearing comfortable slippers or padded socks at home can keep your feet warm, protecting them from draughts of cold air from beneath doors.

Remember a positive moment from this week. Pause and bring it back clearly to your mind. Treasuring moments of happiness not only feels good but it also boosts your immune system.

Self-care is not just about making positive lifestyle choices but also developing healthy relationships. Contact a friend or family member whose company you enjoy. Your well-being will benefit from feeling seen and heard, reminding you that you are not alone.

If you want to fly, you have to give up the things that weigh you down.

TONI MORRISON

In wintertime, heated indoor air can become dry and negatively affect your breathing and skin. You can make your own humidifier to add moisture to the air by filling a heat-safe bowl with water, adding some drops of essential oil (like lavender or geranium oil) and placing it on top of a radiator. When the radiator is on, the water will evaporate, increasing air moisture.

Learn to recognize your own clues when stress is getting too much. This might be snapping at someone, wanting to withdraw socially or going over the same thing in your mind countless times. Take preventative action and give yourself a reset.

Expressing appreciation is a powerful self-care tool in relationships. Using the phrase "Something I appreciate about you is..." will help people around you to think, feel and collaborate better.

To help relax in the evening, soak your feet in warm water for 10 minutes. This increases blood circulation to your feet and legs and reduces swelling. Wipe your feet dry on a soft towel and gently apply moisturizer to your feet, massaging between your toes.

Caring for myself is not self-indulgence, it is self-preservation.

AUDRE LORDE

Be inspired by the ancient Chinese practice of *Yang Sheng* (meaning "nourishing life") to improve your health. Send a smile to each of your organs in turn (your heart, lungs, liver, kidneys and stomach). Take three long, slow breaths; imagine filling each breath with joy and warmth then send the breath to the organ you are focusing on.

Consider where in the world you would love to visit. Let your mind go there. Maybe it is a place you went to a long while ago, or an entirely new place. How might you make it happen?

Candle-gazing is a gentle, tech-free way of meditating. Light a candle in a darkened room, place the candle at arm's length in front of you and focus on the flame. Choose what the flame represents for you. This can help you to develop patience and, in turn, peace.

If you're feeling disappointed about something that matters to you, you don't have to deny your experience. Naming your true feelings will expand your awareness of what you need in this moment.

Try to resist checking your phone first thing in the morning. Allow yourself time to wake up, stretch, feel your feet on the floor and smile. Choose how you want to start your day rather than being dragged into whatever is occurring on your phone.

Everyone feels scared, angry or miserable sometimes. Instead of saying "I am angry" say "I feel angry." Using the word "feel" is less fixed and reminds you that emotions change. Remember that you are not your feelings.

Accept how life is today. Acceptance doesn't mean liking how everything is, that is approval. Let everything be just as it is, in this moment. Smile at what brings you joy. Practising acceptance will help you feel calmer.

Go for a gentle walk. A few minutes of low-intensity movement will activate your metabolism (how your body's cells change food into energy), increasing oxygen to your blood and strengthening your lungs and heart.

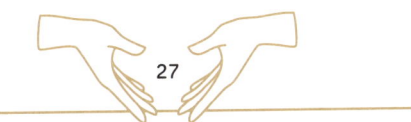

27

At the centre of your being you have the answer; you know who you are and you know what you want.

LAO TZU

Use "box breathing" to stay centred when you feel stressed. Notice a square object, like a window, and count to four as your eyes move along each side of the box. Breathe in as your focus moves across the top edge, then hold your breath as your gaze goes down the first side. Breathe out, counting to four, as your eyes trace the bottom of the square. Then stay with the out breath as your gaze goes up the other side.

Which tips in this book make you think "I'm never doing that!"? That's fine. Self-care isn't about doing what someone else tells you to do. Do the opposite of one of the tips and notice what happens. Or improve them. This is your book, after all.

Zoom out and take stock of where you are. Different stages of life make different demands on your body, energy and resources. Self-care isn't fixed but needs to evolve with you as you grow.

What has been your favourite self-care discovery this year? Perhaps you have reconnected with something meaningful from years ago or have been introduced to something new from elsewhere in the world. Cherish this discovery and take it with you into tomorrow.

conclusion

Another year has come to a close and hopefully you have been able to reflect, consider and take action to care for yourself, inspired by daily entries in this book. How has it felt? What insights have arisen for you on this self-care journey? What is different for you now? Perhaps there were days you remembered and days you forgot. That's okay, you are only human! The good news is that a new year begins tomorrow, and the invitation to deepen your self-care is offered to you once again. Remember, life is precious, and you are a precious expression of life.

also available

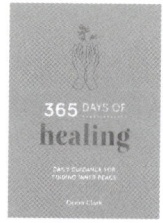

365 DAYS OF HEALING

ISBN: 978-1-83799-373-4

Quinn Clark

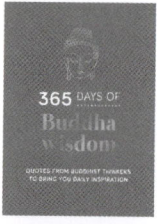

365 DAYS OF
BUDDHA WISDOM

ISBN: 978-1-83799-389-5

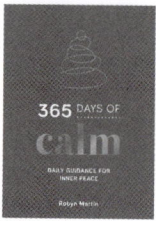

365 DAYS OF CALM

ISBN: 978-1-80007-443-9

Robyn Martin

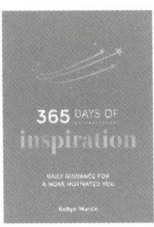

365 DAYS OF INSPIRATION

ISBN: 978-1-80007-444-6

Robyn Martin

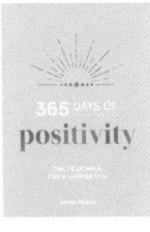

365 DAYS OF POSITIVITY

ISBN: 978-1-80007-102-5

Debbi Marco

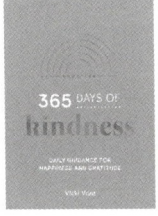

365 DAYS OF KINDNESS

ISBN: 978-1-80007-100-1

Vicki Vrint

Have you enjoyed this book?
If so, find us on Facebook at
Summersdale Publishers, on Twitter/X at
@Summersdale and on Instagram, TikTok
and Bluesky at @summersdalebooks and
get in touch. We'd love to hear from you!

www.summersdale.com